CW00686671

Dear Fiona
get well soon to
your lovable
best.

All
My Love
for
Valentine's
Day 1999

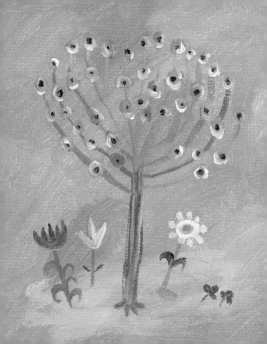

get well

Words to Make You Feel Better

Illustrated by Donna Ingemanson

Ariel Books

Andrews McMeel Publishing

Kansas City

www.andrewsmcmeel.com

ISBN: 0-8362-6798-2
Library of Congress Catalog Card
Number:98-84238

Contents

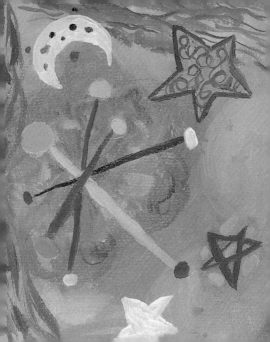

Introduction

The power of heal-
ing is always within
our reach, whether
it's a positive attitude
that gets us through
the day or a simple
quote that reminds us
to enjoy and learn
from everyday life ex-
periences. It has long

been a belief that the mind plays a large role in the healing process. Inspired by words, people can find the strength and fortitude to face and conquer illness.

Gathered here is a collection of quotations from some of the

world's greatest physi-
cians, scientists, and
even humorists. Let
their words be the
powerful elixir that
puts you on the road
to recovery.

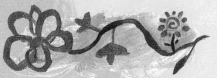

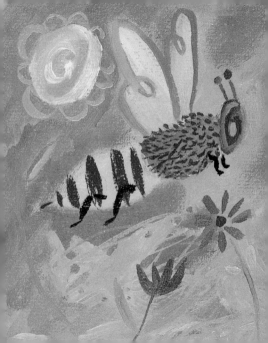

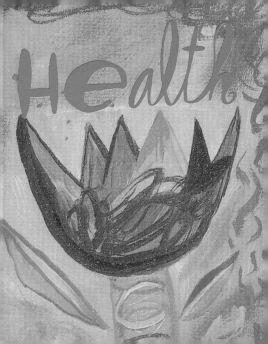

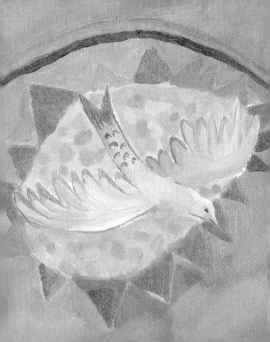

The human body experiences a powerful gravitational pull in the direction of hope. That is why the patient's hopes are the physician's secret weapon. They are hidden ingredients in any prescription.
—NORMAN COUSINS

There's lots of people in this world who spend so much time watching their health, that they haven't the time to enjoy it.

—JOSH BILLINGS

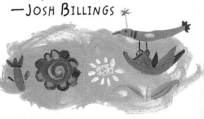

What does not
destroy me, makes
me strong.
— FRIEDRICH NIETZSCHE

Hope! of all ills
that men endure
  The only cheap and
universal cure.
— ABRAHAM COWLEY

Health is the thing
that makes you feel
that now is the best
time of the year.
—FRANKLIN PIERCE
ADAMS

Get Well

16

*N*othing is more desirable than to be released from an affliction, but nothing is more frightening than to be divested of a crutch.

—JAMES BALDWIN

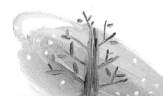

The tongue ever
turns to the aching
tooth.
—PROVERB

The first wealth is
health.
—RALPH WALDO
EMERSON

Get Well

18

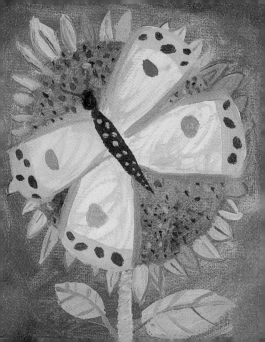

So many people
spend their health
gaining wealth, and
then have to spend
their wealth to regain
their health.
—A. J. REB MATERI

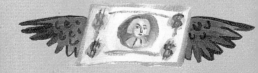

When we are sick
our virtues and vices
are in abeyance.
—VAUVENARGUES

I enjoy convales-
cence. It's the part
that makes illness
worthwhile.
—GEORGE BERNARD
SHAW

Most things
get better by them-
selves. Most things, in
fact, are better by
morning.
—LEWIS THOMAS

22

Long life to you!
Good health to you
and your household!
And good health to
all that is yours!
—I SAMUEL 25:6

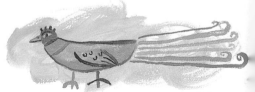

Measure your health by your sympathy with morning and Spring. If there is no response in you to the awakening of nature, if the prospect of an early morning walk does not banish sleep, if the warble of the first bluebird does

not thrill you, you
know that the morn-
ing and spring of your
life are past. Thus may
you feel your pulse.
—HENRY DAVID
    THOREAU

Health

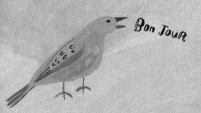
Bon Jour

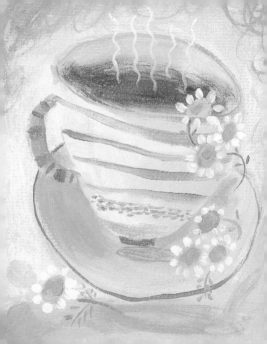

We forget our-
selves and destinies in
health, and the chief
use of temporary
sickness is to remind
us of these concerns.
—RALPH WALDO
    EMERSON

Get Well

In medicine, as in statecraft and propaganda, words are sometimes the most powerful drugs we can use.

—DR. SARA MURRAY JORDAN

28

There is nothing
the body suffers
which the soul may
not profit by.
—GEORGE MEREDITH

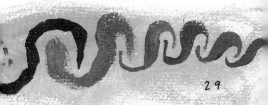

Fight on, my merry men all,
  I'm a little wounded,
but I am not slain;
  I will lay me down
for to bleed a while,
  Then I'll rise and
fight with you again.
—JOHN DRYDEN

30

Positive attitudes—optimism, high self-esteem, an outgoing nature, joyousness, and the ability to cope with stress—may be the most important bases for continued good health.
—HELEN HAYES

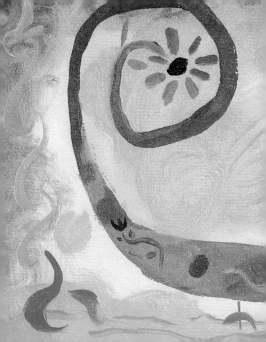

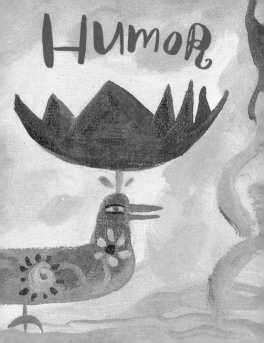

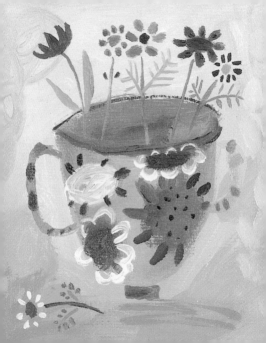

God heals, and the doctor takes the fees.
— BENJAMIN FRANKLIN

If a man thinks about his physical or moral state, he usually discovers that he is ill.
— GOETHE

Doctor, feel my
purse.
—JANE ACE

It's no longer a
question of staying
healthy. It's a ques-
tion of finding a sick-
ness you like.
—JACKIE WILSON

The only way to
keep your health is to
eat what you don't
want, drink what you
don't like, and do
what you'd druther
not.
—MARK TWAIN

Humor

We are usually the
best men when in the
worst health.
— ENGLISH PROVERB

Health consists of
having the same dis-
eases as one's neigh-
bors.
— QUENTIN CRISP

Get Well

38

To avoid delay,
please have all your
symptoms ready.
— NOTICE IN A
  BRITISH DOCTOR'S
  OFFICE

Humor

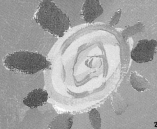

39

Some of the papers presented at today's medical meeting tell us what we already know, but in a much more complicated manner.

— ALPHONSE RAYMOND DOCHEZ

The nurse sleeps
sweetly, hired to
watch the sick,
   Whom, snoring, she
disturbs.
—WILLIAM COWPER

If you look like
your passport photo,
you're too ill to travel.
—WILL KOMMEN

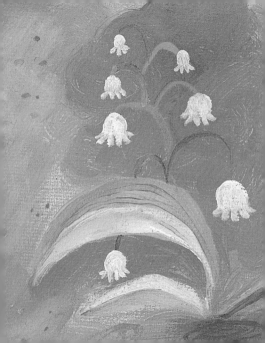

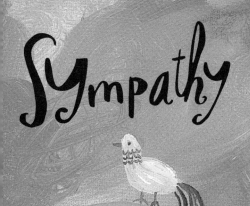

Sympathy

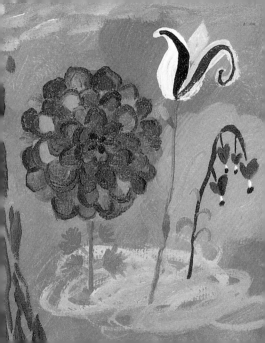

In the sickroom,
ten cents' worth of
human understanding
equals ten dollars'
worth of medical
science.
—MARTIN H. FISCHER

Sympathy

To be sick is to en-
joy monarchal pre-
rogatives.
— CHARLES LAMB

The sorrow which
has no vent in tears
may make other
organs weep.
— HENRY MAUDSLEY

The love of our neighbor in all its fullness simply means being able to say to him, "What are you going through?"
—SIMONE WEIL

I was sick, and ye visited me...
—MATTHEW 25:36

Sympathy

47

Let no one under-
estimate the need of
pity. We live in a stony
universe whose hard,
brilliant forces rage
fiercely.
—THEODORE DREISER

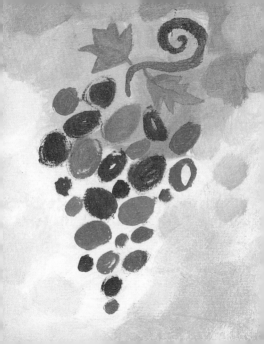

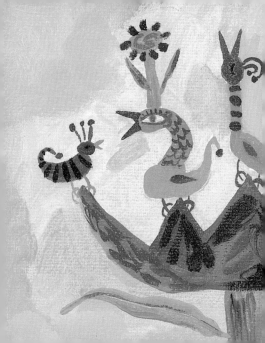

Advice

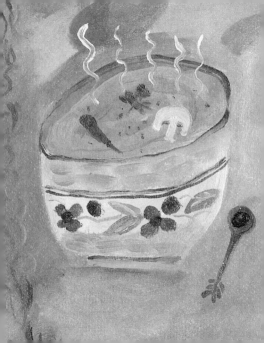

Worries go down
better with soup than
without.
—JEWISH PROVERB

When we are well,
we all have good
advice for those who
are ill.
—TERENCE

Let nothing disturb
thee,
Let nothing affright
thee,
All things are
passing,
God changeth
never.

—HENRY WADSWORTH
LONGFELLOW

54

A good gulp of hot whiskey at bedtime—it's not very scientific, but it helps.
— ALEXANDER D. FLEMING

The remedy against bad times is to have patience with them.
— ARAB PROVERB

B e good to your-
self,
   B e excellent to
others, and
   D o everything with
love.
—JOHN WOLF

Get Well

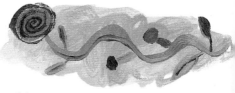

The more serious
the illness, the more
important it is for you
to fight back, mobi-
lizing all your re-
sources—spiritual,
emotional, intellectu-
al, physical.
—NORMAN COUSINS

Advice

I reckon being ill is one of the greatest pleasures of life, provided one is not too ill and is not obliged to work 'til one is better.
—SAMUEL BUTLER

Get Well

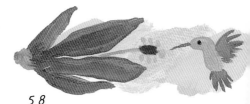

58

A wise man should
consider that health
is the greatest of
human blessings, and
learn how by his own
thought to derive
benefit from his
illnesses.

—HIPPOCRATES

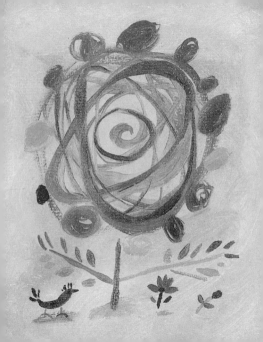

A vigorous five-mile walk will do more good for an unhappy but otherwise healthy adult than all the medicine and psychology in the world.
—PAUL DUDLEY WHITE

Advice

A general flavor
of mild decay,
   But nothing local,
as one may say.
—OLIVER WENDELL
   HOLMES

Wait and see.
—HERBERT HENRY
   ASQUITH

Get Well

62

You gain strength, courage, and confidence by every experience in which you really stop to look fear in the face.... You must do the thing you think you cannot do.

— ELEANOR ROOSEVELT

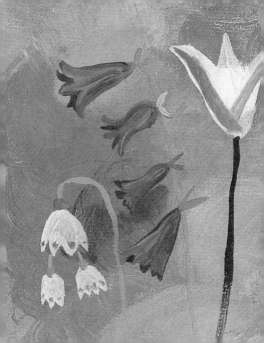

Doctors

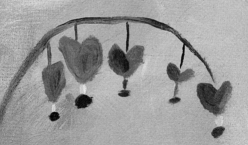

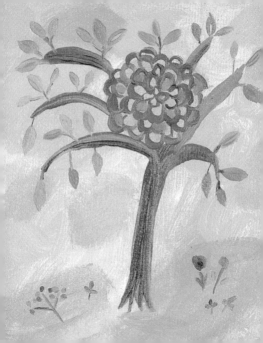

*N*ature, time, and patience are the three great physicians.
—PROVERB

*T*here's nothing wrong with you that an expensive operation can't prolong.
—GRAHAM CHAPMAN

Doctors are busy playing God when so few of us have the qualifications. And besides, the job is taken.

—BERNIE S. SIEGEL, M.D.

Get Well

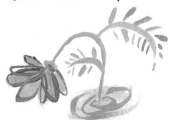

My doctor, Nick the Knife, is a specialist . . . he specializes in cutting up my knees and sticking needles into me. And he's really painless—he doesn't feel any pain at all.

—JOE NAMATH

Common sense is in medicine the master workman.
— PETER LATHAM

Nothing is more fatal to health than an overcare of it.
— BENJAMIN FRANKLIN

*E*very invalid is a
physician.
—IRISH PROVERB

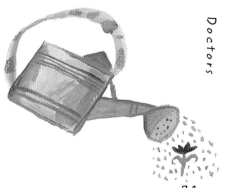

Doctors

71

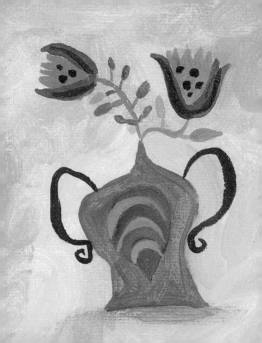

Our doctor would never really operate unless it was necessary. He was just that way. If he didn't need the money, he wouldn't lay a hand on you.
—HERB SHRINER

Doctors

As long as men are liable to die and are desirous to live, a physician will be made fun of, but he will be well paid.

—JEAN DE LA BRUYÈRE

Get Well

74

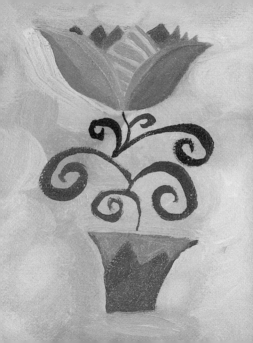

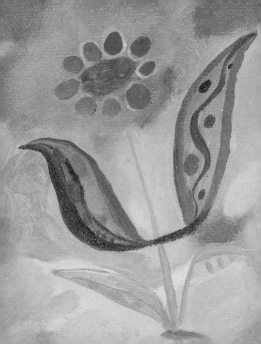

A friend of mine went to the doctor about a ringing in his ear. The doctor gave him an unlisted number.

—CHARLIE CALLAS

Doctors

*N*ever argue with
a doctor; he has in-
side information.
—BOB AND RAY

I observe the
physician with the
same diligence as the
disease.
—JOHN DONNE

*N*ever go to a
doctor whose office
plants are dead.
— ERMA BOMBECK

*N*o doctor takes
pleasure in the health
even of his friends.
— MONTAIGNE

Doctors

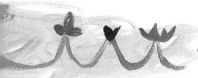

This book was typeset
and designed at
Snap-Haus Graphics
in Edgewater, N.J.

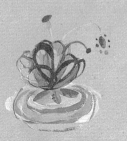